CW01376217

THE MEDITERRANEAN DIET COOKBOOK PORK, BEEF AND POULTRY RECIPES

Quick, Easy and Tasty Recipes to feel full of energy, stay healthy keeping your weight under control

Melanie Castelli

Copyright © 2021 by Melanie Castelli

All right reserved. No part of this publication may be reproduced in any form without permission in writing form the publisher, except for brief quotations used for publishable articles or reviews.

Legal Disclaimer

The information contained in this book and its contents is not designed to replace any form of medical or professional advice; and is not meant to replace the need for independent medical, financial, legal, or other professional advice or service that may require. The content and information in this book have been provided for educational and entertainment purposes only.

The content and information contained in this book have been compiled from sources deemed reliable, and they are accurate to the best of the Author's knowledge, information and belief.

However, the Author cannot guarantee its accuracy and validity and therefore cannot be held liable for any errors and/or omissions.

Further, changes are periodically made to this book as needed. Where appropriate and/or necessary, you must consult a professional (including but not limited to your doctor, attorney, financial advisor, or other such professional) before using any of the suggested remedies, techniques, and/or information in this book.

Upon using this book's contents and information, you agree to hold harmless the Author from any damaged, costs and expenses, including any legal fees potentially resulting from the application of any of the information in this book. This disclaimer applies to any loss, damages, or injury caused by the use and application of this book's content, whether directly and indirectly, whether for breach of contract, tort, negligence, personal injury, criminal intent, or under any other circumstances.

You agree to accept all risks of using the information presented in this book. You agree that by continuing to read this book, where appropriate and/or necessary, you shall consult a professional (including but not limited to your doctor, attorney, financial advisor, or other such professional) before remedies, techniques, and/or information in this book.

The Mediterranean Diet Cookbook: Pork, Beef and Poultry Recipes

The Mediterranean Diet Cookbook: Pork, Beef and Poultry Recipes

TABLE OF CONTENTS

Pressure Cooker Moroccan Pot Roast 8

Shawarma Pork Tenderloin with Pitas 10

Flank Steak with Artichokes 13

Easy Honey-Garlic Pork Chops 15

Moussaka 17

Herbed Lamb Leg 20

Baked Pork Chops 21

Coconut Pork Steaks 22

Beef with Artichokes 23

Beef with Mushrooms & Herbs 24

Ita Sandwiches 25

Shredded Beef 26

Pork Tenderloin & Couscous 27

Braised Lamb Shanks with Veggies 29

Rosemary Baked Lamb 30

Roasted Pork Shoulder 31

Herb Roasted Pork 32

Slow Cooked Beef Brisket 34

Mediterranean Beef Dish 35

Beef Tartar 36

The Mediterranean Diet Cookbook: Pork, Beef and Poultry Recipes

Meatballs and Sauce 37

Rosemary Beef Chuck Roast 39

Herb-Roasted Turkey Breast 41

Chicken Sausage and Peppers 43

Chicken Piccata 45

Chicken with Onions, Potatoes, Figs, and Carrots 47

Chicken Gyros with Tzatziki 49

Greek Chicken Salad 51

One Pot Greek Chicken and Lemon Rice 53

Balsamic Beef Dish 56

Greek Chicken with Vegetables and Lemon Vinaigrette 58

Simple Grilled Salmon with Veggies 60

Caprese Chicken Hasselback Style 62

Grilled Calamari with Lemon Juice 64

Bacon-Wrapped Chicken 66

Broccoli Pesto Spaghetti 68

Creamy Chicken Breasts 70

Cheese Garlic Chicken & Potatoes 72

Easy Chicken Scampi 74

Protein Packed Chicken Bean Rice 75

Pesto Vegetable Chicken 77

Greek Chicken Rice 79

Flavorful Chicken Tacos 81

Quinoa Chicken Bowls 83

Quick Chicken with Mushrooms 85

Herb Garlic Chicken 87

The Mediterranean Diet Cookbook: Pork, Beef and Poultry Recipes

Flavorful Mediterranean Chicken..88

Artichoke Olive Chicken 90

Easy Chicken Piccata 92

Garlic Thyme Chicken Drumsticks 94

Tender Chicken & Mushrooms..96

Delicious Chicken Casserole..98

Perfect Chicken & Rice 100

Moroccan Chicken..102

Flavorful Cafe Rio Chicken 104

Zesty Veggie Chicken..106

Pressure Cooker Moroccan Pot Roast

Preparation time: 15 minutes

Cooking time: 50 minutes

Servings: 4

INGREDIENTS:

- ✓ 8 ounces mushrooms, sliced
- ✓ 4 tablespoons extra-virgin olive oil
- ✓ 3 small onions, cut into 2-inch pieces
- ✓ 2 tablespoons paprika
- ✓ 1½ tablespoons garam masala
- ✓ 2 teaspoons salt
- ✓ ¼ teaspoon ground white pepper
- ✓ 2 tablespoons tomato paste
- ✓ 1 small eggplant, peeled and diced
- ✓ 1¼ cups low-sodium beef broth
- ✓ ½ cup halved apricots
- ✓ 1/3 cup golden raisins
- ✓ 3 pounds beef chuck roast
- ✓ 2 tablespoons honey
- ✓ 1 tablespoon dried mint
- ✓ 2 cups cooked brown rice

DIRECTIONS:

1. Set an electric pressure cooker to Sauté and put the mushrooms and oil in the cooker. Sauté for 5 minutes, then add the onions, paprika, garam masala, salt, and white pepper. Stir in the tomato paste and continue to sauté.
2. Add the eggplant and sauté for 5 more minutes, until softened. Pour in the broth. Add the apricots and raisins. Sear the meat for 2 minutes on each side. Close and lock the lid and set the pressure cooker too high for 50 minutes.
3. When cooking is complete, quick release the pressure. Carefully remove the lid, then remove the meat from the sauce and break it into pieces. While the meat is removed, stir honey and mint into the sauce.
4. Assemble plates with ½ cup of brown rice, ½ cup of pot roast sauce, and 3 to 5 pieces of pot roast.

NUTRITION: Calories: 829 Protein: 69g Carbohydrates: 70g Fat: 34g

Shawarma Pork Tenderloin with Pitas

Preparation time: 15 minutes
Cooking time: 35 minutes
Servings: 8

INGREDIENTS:
- For the shawarma spice rub:
- 1 teaspoon ground cumin
- 1 teaspoon ground coriander
- 1 teaspoon ground turmeric
- ¾ teaspoon sweet Spanish paprika
- ½ teaspoon ground cloves
- ¼ teaspoon salt
- ¼ teaspoon freshly ground black pepper
- 1/8 teaspoon ground cinnamon
- For the shawarma:
- 1½ pounds pork tenderloin
- 3 tablespoons extra-virgin olive oil
- 1 tablespoon garlic powder
- Salt
- Freshly ground black pepper
- 1½ tablespoons Shawarma Spice Rub

The Mediterranean Diet Cookbook: Pork, Beef and Poultry Recipes

- ✓ 4 pita pockets, halved, for serving
- ✓ 1 to 2 tomatoes, sliced, for serving
- ✓ ¼ cup Pickled Onions, for serving
- ✓ ¼ cup Pickled Turnips, for serving
- ✓ ¼ cup store-bought hummus or Garlic-Lemon Hummus

DIRECTIONS:

1. To Make the Shawarma Seasoning:
2. In a small bowl, combine the cumin, coriander, turmeric, paprika, cloves, salt, pepper, and cinnamon and set aside.
3. To Make the Shawarma:
4. Preheat the oven to 400°F. Put the pork tenderloin on a plate and cover with olive oil and garlic powder on each side.
5. Season with salt and pepper and rub each side of the tenderloin with a generous amount of shawarma spices.
6. Place the pork tenderloin in the center of a roasting pan and roast for 20 minutes per pound, or until the meat begins to bounce back as you poke it.
7. If it feels like there's still fluid under the skin, continue cooking. Check every 5 to 7 minutes until

it reaches the desired tenderness and juices run clear.

8. Remove the pork from the oven and let rest for 10 minutes. Serve the pork tenderloin shawarma with pita pockets, tomatoes, Pickled Onions (if using), Pickled Turnips (if using), and hummus.

NUTRITION: Calories: 316 Protein: 29g Carbohydrates: 17g Fat: 15g

The Mediterranean Diet Cookbook: Pork, Beef and Poultry Recipes

Flank Steak with Artichokes

Preparation time: 15 minutes
Cooking time: 60 minutes
Servings: 4-6

INGREDIENTS:

- ✓ 4 tablespoons grapeseed oil, divided
- ✓ 2 pounds flank steak
- ✓ 1 (14-ounce) can artichoke hearts, drained and roughly chopped
- ✓ 1 onion, diced
- ✓ 8 garlic cloves, chopped
- ✓ 1 (32-ounce) container low-sodium beef broth
- ✓ 1 (14.5-ounce) can diced tomatoes, drained
- ✓ 1 cup tomato sauce
- ✓ 2 tablespoons tomato paste
- ✓ 1 teaspoon dried oregano
- ✓ 1 teaspoon dried parsley
- ✓ 1 teaspoon dried basil
- ✓ ½ teaspoon ground cumin
- ✓ 3 bay leaves
- ✓ 2 to 3 cups cooked couscous (optional)

DIRECTIONS:

1. Preheat the oven to 450ºF. In an oven-safe sauté pan or skillet, heat 3 tablespoons of oil on medium heat.
2. Sear the steak for 2 minutes per side on both sides. Transfer the steak to the oven for 30 minutes, or until desired tenderness.
3. Meanwhile, in a large pot, combine the remaining 1 tablespoon of oil, artichoke hearts, onion, and garlic.
4. Pour in the beef broth, tomatoes, tomato sauce, and tomato paste. Stir in oregano, parsley, basil, cumin, and bay leaves.
5. Cook the vegetables, covered, for 30 minutes. Remove bay leaf and serve with flank steak and ½ cup of couscous per plate, if using.

NUTRITION: Calories: 577 Protein: 55g Carbohydrates: 22g Fat: 28g

Easy Honey-Garlic Pork Chops

Preparation time: 15 minutes
Cooking time: 25 minutes
Servings: 4

INGREDIENTS:

- 4 pork chops, boneless or bone-in
- ¼ teaspoon salt
- 1/8 teaspoon freshly ground black pepper
- 3 tablespoons extra-virgin olive oil
- 5 tablespoons low-sodium chicken broth, divided
- 6 garlic cloves, minced
- ¼ cup honey
- 2 tablespoons apple cider vinegar

DIRECTIONS:

1. Season the pork chops with salt and pepper and set aside.
2. In a large sauté pan or skillet, heat the oil over medium-high heat. Add the pork chops and sear for 5 minutes on each side, or until golden brown.
3. Once the searing is complete, move the pork to a dish and reduce the skillet heat from medium-high to medium.

4. Add 3 tablespoons of chicken broth to the pan; this will loosen the bits and flavors from the bottom of the skillet.
5. Once the broth has evaporated, add the garlic to the skillet and cook for 15 to 20 seconds, until fragrant.
6. Add the honey, vinegar, and the remaining 2 tablespoons of broth. Bring the heat back up to medium-high and continue to cook for 3 to 4 minutes.
7. Stir periodically; the sauce is ready once it's thickened slightly. Add the pork chops back into the pan, cover them with the sauce, and cook for 2 minutes. Serve.

NUTRITION: Calories: 302 Protein: 22g Carbohydrates: 19g Fat: 16g

Moussaka

Preparation time: 15 minutes
Cooking time: 40 minutes
Servings: 6-8

INGREDIENTS:

- For the eggplant:
- 2 pounds eggplant, cut into ¼-inch-thick slices
- 1 teaspoon salt
- 2 to 3 tablespoons extra-virgin olive oil
- For the filling:
- 1 tablespoon extra-virgin olive oil
- 2 shallots, diced
- 1 tablespoon dried, minced garlic
- 1 pound ground lamb
- 4 ounces portobello mushrooms, diced
- 1 (14.5-ounce) can crushed tomatoes, drained
- ¼ cup tomato paste
- 1 cup low-sodium beef broth
- 2 bay leaves
- 2 teaspoons dried oregano
- ¾ teaspoon salt

The Mediterranean Diet Cookbook: Pork, Beef and Poultry Recipes

- ✓ 2½ cups store-bought béchamel sauce
- ✓ 1/3 cup panko bread crumbs

DIRECTIONS:

1. To Make the Eggplant
2. Preheat the oven to 450°F. Line large baking sheets with paper towels and arrange the eggplant slices in a single layer and sprinkle with salt.
3. Place another layer of paper towel on the eggplant slices. Continue until all eggplant slices are covered.
4. Let the eggplant sweat for 30 minutes to remove excess moisture. While this is happening, make the meat sauce.
5. Pat the eggplant dry. Dry the baking sheets and brush with oil and place the eggplant slices onto the baking sheets.
6. Bake for 15 to 20 minutes, or until lightly browned and softened. Remove from the oven and cool slightly before assembling the moussaka.
7. In a large, oven-safe sauté pan or skillet, heat the olive oil over high heat. Cook the shallots and garlic for 2 minutes, until starting to soften.
8. Add the ground lamb and brown it with the garlic and onions, breaking it up as it cooks.

9. Add the mushrooms and cook for 5 to 7 minutes, or until they have dehydrated slightly.
10. Add the tomatoes and paste, beef broth, bay leaves, oregano, and salt and stir to combine
11. Once the sauce is simmering, lower to medium-low and cook for 15 minutes, or until it reduces to a thick sauce.
12. Remove the sauce to a separate bowl before assembly. Reduce the oven temperature to 350°F.
13. Place half the eggplant slices in the bottom of the skillet used to make the sauce. Top the slices with all the meat filling.
14. Place the remaining eggplant on top of the meat filling and pour the jarred béchamel sauce over the eggplant. Sprinkle with the bread crumbs.Bake for 30 to 40 minutes or until golden brown. Let stand for 10 minutes before serving.

NUTRITION: Calories: 491 Protein: 23g Carbohydrates: 30g Fat: 33g

Herbed Lamb Leg

Preparation time: 15 minutes

Cooking time: 50 Minutes

Servings: 4

INGREDIENTS:

- ✓ 1 1/2-pound lamb leg, trimmed, meat only
- ✓ 1 tablespoon Provance herbs
- ✓ 1 teaspoon salt
- ✓ 1 tablespoon olive oil

DIRECTIONS:

1. Rub the lamb led with Provance herbs and salt. Then brush it carefully with olive oil and wrap in the foil.
2. Bake the meat for 50 minutes at 360F. Then discard the foil and chill the lamb meat little. Slice it.

NUTRITION: Calories 336 Fat 14.9g Carbs 0g Protein 47.9g

Baked Pork Chops

Preparation time: 15 minutes
Cooking time: 30 Minutes
Servings: 4

INGREDIENTS:
- 4 pork loin chops, boneless
- A pinch of salt and black pepper
- 1 tablespoon sweet paprika
- 2 tablespoons Dijon mustard
- Cooking spray

DIRECTIONS:
1. In a bowl, mix the pork chops with salt, pepper, paprika and the mustard and rub well.
2. Grease a baking sheet with cooking spray, add the pork chops, cover with tin foil, introduce in the oven and bake at 400 degrees F for 30 minutes.
3. Divide the pork chops between plates and serve with a side salad.

NUTRITION: Calories 167 Fat 5g Carbs 2g Protein 25g

Coconut Pork Steaks

Preparation time: 15 minutes

Cooking time: 10 Minutes

Servings: 4

INGREDIENTS:

- ✓ 4 pork steaks (3.5 oz each steak)
- ✓ 1 tablespoon ground turmeric
- ✓ 1 teaspoon salt
- ✓ 1 tablespoon coconut oil
- ✓ 1 teaspoon apple cider vinegar

DIRECTIONS:

1. Rub the pork steaks with ground turmeric, salt, and apple cider vinegar. Melt the coconut oil in the skillet and add pork steaks.
2. Roast the pork steaks for 5 minutes from each side. Serve.

NUTRITION: Calories 366 Fat 28.6g Carbs 2.1g Protein 25.1g

Beef with Artichokes

Preparation time: 15 minutes

Cooking time: 7 Hours And 4 Minutes

Servings: 4

INGREDIENTS:

- ✓ 2 lb. stew beef
- ✓ 14 oz. artichoke hearts, drained and sliced in half
- ✓ 2 tablespoons onion and garlic, minced
- ✓ 32 oz. beef broth
- ✓ 15 oz. tomato sauce

DIRECTIONS:

1. Pour 1 tablespoon oil into the Instant Pot. Set it to sauté. Cook the beef for 2 minutes per side. Cover the pot. Set it to slow cook and set it to 7 hours.

NUTRITION: Calories 505 Fat 19g Carbohydrate 24.8g Protein 60.6g

Beef with Mushrooms & Herbs

Preparation time: 15 minutes

Cooking time: 8 Hours And 5 Minutes

Servings: 6

INGREDIENTS:

- ✓ 1/2 cup garlic cloves, sliced
- ✓ 1 cup mushrooms
- ✓ 2 lb. beef chuck steak, sliced into cubes
- ✓ 1 cup tomatoes with tomato sauce
- ✓ 4 tablespoons mixed dried herbs (rosemary, sage, and parsley)

DIRECTIONS:

1. Pour 1 tablespoon olive oil into the Instant Pot. Add the onion and mushrooms and cook for 5 minutes. Add the beef and cook until brown on both sides.
2. Pour in the rest of the ingredients. Season with salt and pepper. Seal the pot. Set it to slow cook. Cook for 8 hours.

NUTRITION: Calories 400 Fat 17g Carbohydrate 11.9g Protein 48.8g

Ita Sandwiches

Preparation time: 15 minutes
Cooking time: 20 Minutes
Servings: 1 Pita Sandwich

INGREDIENTS:
- 1 lb. ground beef
- 1 tsp. salt
- 1/2 tsp. ground black pepper
- 1 tsp. seven spices
- 4 (6- or 7-in.) pitas

DIRECTIONS:
1. Preheat the oven to 400ºF. In a medium bowl, combine beef, salt, black pepper, and seven spices.
2. Lay out pitas on the counter, and divide beef mixture evenly among them, and spread beef to edge of pitas.
3. Place pitas on a baking sheet, and bake for 20 minutes. Serve warm with Greek yogurt.

NUTRITION: Calories 505 Fat 19g Carbohydrate 24.8g Protein 60.6g

Shredded Beef

Preparation time: 15 minutes
Cooking time: 20 Minutes
Servings: 8

INGREDIENTS:

- ✓ 2 lb. beef chuck roast
- ✓ 1 cup onion, chopped
- ✓ 1 cup mixed frozen vegetables (carrots, bell pepper), chopped
- ✓ 14 oz. canned fire roasted tomatoes
- ✓ 2 tablespoons red wine vinegar

DIRECTIONS:

1. Season the beef with salt. Add to the Instant Pot. Top with the onion and frozen vegetables. Pour the tomatoes and vinegar. Mix well.
2. Seal the pot. Choose manual setting. Cook at high pressure for 20 minutes. Release the pressure quickly. Let cool for 5 minutes. Shred the beef. Season with salt and pepper or Italian blend seasoning.

NUTRITION: Calories 431 Fat 31.6g Carbohydrate 4.3g Protein 30.2g

Pork Tenderloin & Couscous

Preparation time: 15 minutes
Cooking time: 2 Hours And 15 Minutes
Servings: 4

INGREDIENTS:
- 4 cloves garlic, minced and divided
- 1 tablespoon garam masala
- 24 oz. pork tenderloin, minced
- 1 cup couscous
- Dressing (mixture of 1/2 cup olive oil, 2 tablespoons red wine vinegar and 1/2 cup fresh parsley, minced)

DIRECTIONS:
1. Mix the chicken broth and half of the garlic. Pour into the Instant Pot. In a bowl, mix the garam masala with a pinch of salt and pepper.
2. Season the pork with this mixture. Put the pork inside the pot. Cover the pot. Set it to slow cook. Cook for 2 hours. Transfer the pork to a plate and cover with foil.
3. Pour the cooking liquid in a bowl, leaving only 1 cup in the pot. Add the couscous. Cover the pot. Set it to manual. Cook at high pressure for 15 minutes.

4. Release the pressure quickly. Fluff the couscous. Serve the pork with the couscous and dressing.

NUTRITION: Calories 763 Fat 37.9g Carbohydrate 52.2g Protein 54.8g

Braised Lamb Shanks with Veggies

Preparation time: 15 minutes
Cooking time: 28 minutes
Servings: 6

INGREDIENTS:

- 6 lamb shanks
- 1 onion, chopped
- 1 lb. frozen carrots and potatoes, chopped
- Seasoning mixture (2 1/4 teaspoons garlic powder, 1 teaspoon sweet Spanish paprika and 3/4 teaspoon ground nutmeg)
- 28 oz. canned tomatoes with juice

DIRECTIONS:

1. Season the lamb shanks with the seasoning mixture. Pour 2 tablespoons olive oil into the Instant Pot. Set it to sauté.
2. Brown the lamb shanks for 8 minutes. Add the rest of the ingredients. Mix well. Cover the pot. Set it to manual. Cook at high pressure for 20 minutes. Release the pressure naturally.

NUTRITION: Calories 839 Fat 29.9g Carbohydrate 26.6g Protein 97.5g

Rosemary Baked Lamb

Preparation time: 15 minutes

Cooking time: 40 Minutes

Servings: 5

INGREDIENTS:

- 1.5-pound rack of lamb, trimmed
- 1 teaspoon dried rosemary
- 2 tablespoons olive oil
- 1 teaspoon salt

DIRECTIONS:

1. Whisk together olive oil, salt, and dried rosemary. Brush the rack of lamb with the rosemary mixture and wrap in the foil.
2. Bake the rack of lamb for 40 minutes at 360F Then discard the foil and cut the meat on the servings.

NUTRITION: Calories 278 Fat 17.7g Carbs 0.2g Protein 27.7g

Roasted Pork Shoulder

Preparation time: 30 minutes
Cooking time: 4 hours
Servings: 6

INGREDIENTS:

- ✓ 3 tablespoons garlic, minced
- ✓ 3 tablespoons olive oil
- ✓ 4 pounds pork shoulder
- ✓ Salt and black pepper to taste

DIRECTIONS:

1. In a bowl, mix olive oil with salt, pepper and oil and whisk well. Brush pork shoulder with this mix, arrange in a baking dish and place in the oven at 425 degrees for 20 minutes.
2. Reduce heat to 325 degrees F and bake for 4 hours. Take pork shoulder out of the oven, slice and arrange on a platter. Serve with your favorite Mediterranean side salad.

NUTRITION: Calories 224 Fat 31g Carbs 21g Protein 23g

Herb Roasted Pork

Preparation time: 20 minutes
Cooking time: 2 hours
Servings: 10

INGREDIENTS:

- ✓ 5 and ½ pounds pork loin roast, trimmed, chine bone removed
- ✓ Salt and black pepper to taste
- ✓ 3 garlic cloves, minced
- ✓ 2 tablespoons rosemary, chopped
- ✓ 1 teaspoon fennel, ground
- ✓ 1 tablespoon fennel seeds
- ✓ 2 teaspoons red pepper, crushed
- ✓ ¼ cup olive oil

DIRECTIONS:

1. In a food processor mix garlic with fennel seeds, fennel, rosemary, red pepper, some black pepper and the olive oil and blend until you obtain a paste.
2. Place pork roast in a roasting pan, spread 2 tablespoons garlic paste all over and rub well. Season with salt and pepper, place in the oven at 400 degrees F and bake for 1 hour.

3. Reduce heat to 325 degrees F and bake for another 35 minutes. Carve roast into chops, divide between plates and serve right away.

NUTRITION: Calories 320 Fat 31g Carbs 21g Protein 23g

Slow Cooked Beef Brisket

Preparation time: 10 minutes
Cooking time: 9 hours
Servings: 8

INGREDIENTS:

- ✓ 6 pounds beef brisket
- ✓ 2 tablespoons cumin, ground
- ✓ 3 tablespoons rosemary, chopped
- ✓ 2 tablespoons coriander, dried
- ✓ 1 tablespoon oregano, dried
- ✓ 2 teaspoons cinnamon powder
- ✓ 1 cup beef stock
- ✓ A pinch of salt and black pepper

DIRECTIONS:

1. In a slow cooker, combine the beef with the cumin, rosemary, coriander, oregano, cinnamon, salt, pepper and stock. Cover and cook on low for 9 hours. Slice and serve.

NUTRITION: Calories 400 Fat 31g Carbs 21g Protein 23g

Mediterranean Beef Dish

Preparation time: 10 minutes
Cooking time: 15 minutes
Servings: 6

INGREDIENTS:

- 1-pound beef, ground
- 2 cups zucchinis, chopped
- ½ cup yellow onion, chopped Salt and black pepper to taste
- 15 ounces canned roasted tomatoes and garlic
- 1 cup water , ¾ cup cheddar cheese, shredded
- 1 and ½ cups white rice

DIRECTIONS:

1. Heat a pan over medium high heat, add beef, onion, salt, pepper and zucchini, stir and cook for 7 minutes.
2. Add water, tomatoes and garlic, stir and bring to a boil. Add rice, more salt and pepper, stir, cover, take off heat and leave aside for 7 minutes. Divide between plates and serve with cheddar cheese on top.

NUTRITION: Calories 320 Fat 31g Carbs 21g Protein 23g

Beef Tartar

Preparation time: 10 minutes
Cooking time: 0 minutes
Servings: 1

INGREDIENTS:

- ✓ 1 shallot, chopped
- ✓ 4 ounces beef fillet, minced
- ✓ 5 small cucumbers, chopped
- ✓ 1 egg yolk
- ✓ A pinch of salt and black pepper
- ✓ 2 teaspoons mustard
- ✓ 1 tablespoon parsley, chopped
- ✓ 1 parsley spring, roughly chopped for serving

DIRECTIONS:

1. In a bowl, mix meat with shallot, egg yolk, salt, pepper, mustard, cucumbers and parsley. Stir well and arrange on a platter. Garnish with the chopped parsley spring and serve.

NUTRITION: Calories 244 Fat 31g Carbs 21g Protein 23g

Meatballs and Sauce

Preparation time: 5 minutes
Cooking time: 8 minutes
Servings: 4

INGREDIENTS:

- ✓ 1 egg, whisked
- ✓ 1 teaspoon cumin, ground
- ✓ 1 teaspoon allspice, ground
- ✓ ¼ cup cilantro, chopped
- ✓ A pinch of salt and black pepper
- ✓ 2 pounds beef, ground
- ✓ 1/3 cup breadcrumbs
- ✓ Vegetable oil for frying
- ✓ For the sauce:
- ✓ 1 cucumber, chopped
- ✓ 1 cup Greek yogurt
- ✓ 2 tablespoons lemon juice
- ✓ 1 tablespoon dill, chopped

DIRECTIONS:

1. In a bowl, mix the beef with the breadcrumbs, egg, cumin, allspice, cilantro, salt and pepper. Stir well

and shape into medium sized meatballs. Heat a pan with oil over medium heat.

2. Add the meatballs and cook for 4 minutes each side. In a bowl, mix the yogurt with the cucumber, lemon juice and dill - whisk well. Serve the meatballs with the yogurt sauce.

NUTRITION: Calories 263 Fat 31g Carbs 21g Protein 23g

Rosemary Beef Chuck Roast

Preparation time: 5 minutes

Cooking time: 45 minutes

Servings: 5-6

INGREDIENTS:

- ✓ 3 pounds chuck beef roast
- ✓ 3 garlic cloves
- ✓ ¼ cup balsamic vinegar
- ✓ 1 sprig fresh rosemary
- ✓ 1 sprig fresh thyme
- ✓ 1 cup of water
- ✓ 1 tablespoon vegetable oil
- ✓ Salt and pepper to taste

DIRECTIONS:

1. Chop slices in the beef roast and place the garlic cloves in them. Rub the roast with the herbs, black pepper, and salt.
2. Preheat your instant pot using the sauté setting and pour the oil. When warmed, mix in the beef roast and stir-cook until browned on all sides.
3. Add the remaining ingredients; stir gently.

4. Seal tight and cook on high for 40 minutes using manual setting. Allow the pressure release naturally, about 10 minutes. Uncover and put the beef roast the serving plates, slice and serve.

NUTRITION: 542 Calories 11.2g Fat 8.7g Carbohydrates 55.2g Protein 710mg Sodium

Herb-Roasted Turkey Breast

Preparation time: 15 minutes

Cooking time: 1½ hours (plus 20 minutes to rest)

Servings: 2

INGREDIENTS:

- ✓ 2 tablespoons extra-virgin olive oil
- ✓ 4 garlic cloves, minced
- ✓ Zest of 1 lemon
- ✓ 1 tablespoon chopped fresh thyme leaves
- ✓ 1 tablespoon chopped fresh rosemary leaves
- ✓ 2 tablespoons chopped fresh Italian parsley leaves
- ✓ 1 teaspoon ground mustard
- ✓ 1 teaspoon sea salt
- ✓ ¼ teaspoon freshly ground black pepper
- ✓ 1 (6-pound) bone-in, skin-on turkey breast
- ✓ 1 cup dry white wine

DIRECTIONS:

1. Preheat the oven to 325°F. Combine the olive oil, garlic, lemon zest, thyme, rosemary, parsley, mustard, sea salt, and pepper.

2. Brush the herb mixture evenly over the surface of the turkey breast, and loosen the skin and rub underneath as well. Situate the turkey breast in a roasting pan on a rack, skin-side up.
3. Pour the wine in the pan. Roast for 1 to 1½ hours until the turkey reaches an internal temperature of 165 degrees F.
4. Pull out from the oven and set separately for 20 minutes, tented with aluminum foil to keep it warm, before carving.

NUTRITION: 392 Calories 1g Fat 2g Carbohydrates 84g Protein 741mg Sodium

Chicken Sausage and Peppers

Preparation time: 10 minutes
Cooking time: 20 minutes

Servings: 2

INGREDIENTS:

- ✓ 2 tablespoons extra-virgin olive oil
- ✓ 6 Italian chicken sausage links
- ✓ 1 onion
- ✓ 1 red bell pepper
- ✓ 1 green bell pepper
- ✓ 3 garlic cloves, minced
- ✓ ½ cup dry white wine
- ✓ ½ teaspoon sea salt
- ✓ ¼ teaspoon freshly ground black pepper
- ✓ Pinch red pepper flakes

DIRECTIONS:

1. Cook the olive oil on large skillet until it shimmers. Add the sausages and cook for 5 to 7 minutes, turning occasionally, until browned, and they reach an internal temperature of 165°F.

2. With tongs, remove the sausage from the pan and set aside on a platter, tented with aluminum foil to keep warm.
3. Return the skillet to the heat and mix in the onion, red bell pepper, and green bell pepper. Cook and stir occasionally, until the vegetables begin to brown.
4. Put in the garlic and cook for 30 seconds, stirring constantly.
5. Stir in the wine, sea salt, pepper, and red pepper flakes. Pull out and fold in any browned bits from the bottom of the pan.
6. Simmer for about 4 minutes more, stirring, until the liquid reduces by half. Spoon the peppers over the sausages and serve.

NUTRITION: 173 Calories 1g Fat 6g Carbohydrates 22g Protein 582mg Sodium

Chicken Piccata

Preparation time: 10 minutes

Cooking time: 15 minutes

Servings: 2

INGREDIENTS:

- ½ cup whole-wheat flour
- ½ teaspoon sea salt
- 1/8 teaspoon freshly ground black pepper
- 1½ pounds chicken breasts, cut into 6 pieces
- 3 tablespoons extra-virgin olive oil
- 1 cup unsalted chicken broth
- ½ cup dry white wine
- Juice of 1 lemon
- Zest of 1 lemon
- ¼ cup capers, drained and rinsed
- ¼ cup chopped fresh parsley leaves

DIRECTIONS:

- In a shallow dish, whisk the flour, sea salt, and pepper. Scour the chicken in the flour and tap off any excess. Cook the olive oil until it shimmers.

- Put the chicken and cook for about 4 minutes per side until browned. Pull out the chicken from the pan and set aside, tented with aluminum foil to keep warm.
- Situate the skillet back to the heat and stir in the broth, wine, lemon juice, lemon zest, and capers. Use the side of a spoon scoop and fold in any browned bits from the pan's bottom.
- Simmer until the liquid thickens. Take out the skillet from the heat and take the chicken back to the pan. Turn to coat. Stir in the parsley and serve.

NUTRITION: 153 Calories 2g Fat 9g Carbohydrates 8g Protein 692mg Sodium

Chicken with Onions, Potatoes, Figs, and Carrots

Preparation time: 5 minutes

Cooking time: 45 minutes

Servings: 2

INGREDIENTS:

- ✓ 2 cups fingerling potatoes, halved
- ✓ 4 fresh figs, quartered
- ✓ 2 carrots, julienned
- ✓ 2 tablespoons extra-virgin olive oil
- ✓ 1 teaspoon sea salt, divided
- ✓ ¼ teaspoon freshly ground black pepper
- ✓ 4 chicken leg-thigh quarters
- ✓ 2 tablespoons chopped fresh parsley leaves

DIRECTIONS:

1. Preheat the oven to 425°F. In a small bowl, toss the potatoes, figs, and carrots with the olive oil, ½ teaspoon of sea salt, and the pepper. Spread in a 9-by-13-inch baking dish.
2. Season the chicken with the rest of t sea salt. Place it on top of the vegetables. Bake until the

vegetables are soft and the chicken reaches an internal temperature of 165°F.
3. Sprinkle with the parsley and serve.

NUTRITION: 429 Calories 4g Fat 27g Carbohydrates 52g Protein 581mg Sodium

Chicken Gyros with Tzatziki

Preparation time: 15 minutes

Cooking time: 1 hours and 20 minutes

Servings: 2

INGREDIENTS:

- ✓ 1-pound ground chicken breast
- ✓ 1 onion, grated with excess water wrung out
- ✓ 2 tablespoons dried rosemary
- ✓ 1 tablespoon dried marjoram
- ✓ 6 garlic cloves, minced
- ✓ ½ teaspoon sea salt
- ✓ ¼ teaspoon freshly ground black pepper
- ✓ Tzatziki Sauce

DIRECTIONS:

1. Preheat the oven to 350°F. Mix the chicken, onion, rosemary, marjoram, garlic, sea salt, and pepper using food processor.
2. Blend until the mixture forms a paste. Alternatively, mix these ingredients in a bowl until well combined (see preparation tip).
3. Press the mixture into a loaf pan. Bake until it reaches 165 degrees internal temperature. Take

out from the oven and let rest for 20 minutes before slicing.
4. Slice the gyro and spoon the tzatziki sauce over the top.

NUTRITION: 289 Calories 1g Fat 20g Carbohydrates 50g Protein 622mg Sodium

Greek Chicken Salad

Preparation time: 15 minutes

Cooking time: 30 minutes

Servings: 2

INGREDIENTS:

- ✓ 1/4 cup balsamic vinegar
- ✓ 1 teaspoon freshly squeezed lemon juice
- ✓ 1/4 cup extra-virgin olive oil
- ✓ 1/4 teaspoon salt
- ✓ 1/4 teaspoon freshly ground black pepper
- ✓ 2 grilled boneless, skinless chicken breasts, sliced (about 1 cup)
- ✓ 1/2 cup thinly sliced red onion
- ✓ 10 cherry tomatoes, halved
- ✓ 8 pitted Kalamata olives, halved
- ✓ 2 cups roughly chopped romaine lettuce
- ✓ 1/2 cup feta cheese

DIRECTIONS:

1. In a medium bowl, combine the vinegar and lemon juice and stir well. Slowly whisk in the olive oil and

continue whisking vigorously until well blended. Whisk in the salt and pepper.
2. Add the chicken, onion, tomatoes, and olives and stir well. Cover and refrigerate for at least 2 hours or overnight.
3. To serve, divide the romaine between 2 salad plates and top each with half of the chicken vegetable mixture. Top with feta cheese and serve immediately.

NUTRITION: 173 Calories 1g Fat 6g Carbohydrates 22g Protein 582mg Sodium

The Mediterranean Diet Cookbook: Pork, Beef and Poultry Recipes

One Pot Greek Chicken and Lemon Rice

Preparation time: 15 minutes
Cooking time: 30 minutes
Servings: 20
INGREDIENTS:

- ✓ Chicken and Marinade
- ✓ 5 chicken thighs, skin on, bone in (about 1 kg / 2 lb.) (Note 1)
- ✓ 1 - 2 lemons, use the zest + 4 tbsp lemon juice (Note 7)
- ✓ 1 tbsp dried oregano
- ✓ 4 garlic cloves, minced
- ✓ 1/2 tsp salt

   1. Rice

- ✓ 1 1/2 tbsp olive oil, separated
- ✓ 1 small onion, finely diced
- ✓ 1 cup (180g) long grain rice, uncooked (Note 6)
- ✓ 1 1/2 cups (375 ml) chicken broth / stock
- ✓ 3/4 cup (185 ml) water
- ✓ 1 tbsp dried oregano
- ✓ 3/4 tsp salt

- ✓ Black pepper

2. Garnish

- ✓ Finely chopped parsley or oregano (optional)
- ✓ Fresh lemon zest (highly recommended)

DIRECTIONS:

1. Combine the Chicken and Marinade ingredients in a Ziplock bag and set aside for at least 20 minutes but preferably overnight.
2. TO COOK
3. Preheat oven to 180°C/350°F.
4. Remove chicken from marinade, but reserve the Marinade.
5. Heat 1/2 tbsp olive oil in a deep, heavy based skillet (Note 2) over medium high heat.
6. Place the chicken in the skillet, skin side down, and cook until golden brown, then turn and cook the other side until golden brown.
7. Remove the chicken and set aside.
8. Pour off fat and wipe the pan with a scrunched-up ball of paper towel (to remove black bits), then return to the stove.
9. Heat 1 tbsp olive oil in the skillet over medium high heat. Add the onion and sauté for a few minutes until translucent.

10. Then add the remaining Rice ingredients and reserved Marinade.
11. Let the liquid come to a simmer and let it simmer for 30 seconds. Place the chicken on top then place a lid on the skillet (Note 3).
12. Bake in the oven for 35 minutes. Then remove the lid and bake for a further 10 minutes, or until all the liquid is absorbed and the rice is tender (so 45 minutes in total)
13. Remove from the oven and allow to rest for 5 to 10 minutes before serving, garnished with parsley or oregano and fresh lemon zest, if desired.

NUTRITION: 173 Calories 1g Fat 6g Carbohydrates 22g Protein 582mg Sodium

Balsamic Beef Dish

Preparation time: 15 minutes

Cooking time: 45 minutes

Servings: 2

INGREDIENTS:

- ✓ 3 lbs. or 1360 g chuck roast
- ✓ 3 cloves garlic, sliced
- ✓ 1 tbsp. oil
- ✓ 1 tsp. flavored vinegar
- ✓ ½ tsp. pepper
- ✓ ½ tsp. rosemary
- ✓ 1 tbsp. butter
- ✓ ½ tsp. thyme
- ✓ 1 c. beef broth

DIRECTIONS:

1. Slice-slit openings in the roast and stuff them with garlic slices.
2. Using a bowl, combine pepper, vinegar, and rosemary. Rub all over the roast.
3. Place your pot on heat. Add in oil and heat on sauté mode.

4. Add in the roast and cook until both sides brown (each side to take 5 minutes). Remove from pot and set aside.
5. Add in thyme, broth, butter, and deglaze your pot.
6. Set back the roast and cook for 40 minutes on High heat while covered.
7. Remove the lid and serve!

NUTRITION: Calories 393, Fat 15 g, Sat. fat 6 g, Fiber 11 g, Carbs 25 g, Sugars 8 g, Protein 37 g, Sodium 438mg

Greek Chicken with Vegetables and Lemon Vinaigrette

Preparation time: 15 minutes

Cooking time: 50 minutes

Servings: 2

INGREDIENTS:

- ✓ For the lemon vinaigrette
- ✓ 1 tsp. lemon zest
- ✓ 1 tbsp. lemon juice
- ✓ 1 tbsp. olive oil
- ✓ 1 tbsp. crumbled feta cheese
- ✓ ½ tsp. honey
- ✓ For the Greek Chicken and roasted veggies
- ✓ 8 oz. or 226.7g boneless chicken breast, skinless and halved
- ✓ ¼ c. light mayonnaise
- ✓ 2 cloves minced garlic
- ✓ ½ c. panko bread crumbs
- ✓ 3 tbsps. Parmesan cheese, grated
- ✓ ½ tsp. kosher salt
- ✓ ½ tsp. black pepper

- ✓ 1 tbsp. olive oil
- ✓ ½ c. dill sliced

DIRECTIONS:

1. To make the vinaigrette, put a teaspoon of zest, one tablespoon of lemon juice, olive oil, cheese, and honey in a bowl.
2. For the vegetables and chicken, preheat the oven to 470 F/243 C. Use a meat mallet for flattening the chicken to two pieces.
3. Using a bowl, set in the chicken. Add in two garlic cloves and mayonnaise. Mix cheese, bread crumbs, pepper, and salt together. Dip the chicken in this crumb mix. Spray olive oil over the chicken.
4. Roast in the oven till the chicken is done and vegetables are tender. Sprinkle dill over it and serve.

NUTRITION: Calories 306, Fat 15 g, Sat. fat 3 g, Fiber 2 g, Carbs 12 g, Sugar 4 g, Protein 30 g, Sodium 432 mg

Simple Grilled Salmon with Veggies

Preparation time: 10 minutes
Cooking time: 25 minutes
Servings: 2

INGREDIENTS:

- 1 halved zucchini
- 2 trimmed oranges, red or yellow bell peppers, halved and seeded
- 1 red onion, wedged
- 1 tbsp. olive oil
- ½ tsp. salt and ground pepper
- 1¼ lbs. or 0.57kg salmon fillet, 4 slices
- ¼ c. sliced fresh basil
- 1 lemon, wedged

DIRECTIONS:

1. Preheat the grill to medium-high. Brush peppers, zucchini, and onion with oil. Sprinkle a ¼ teaspoon of salt over it. Sprinkle salmon with salt and pepper.
2. Place the veggies and the salmon on the grill. Cook the veggies for six to eight minutes on each side,

till the grill marks appear. Cook the salmon till it flakes when you test it with a fork.
3. When cooled down, chop the veggies roughly and mix them in a bowl. You can remove the salmon skin to serve with the veggies.
4. Each serving can be garnished with a tablespoon of basil and a lemon wedge.

NUTRITION: Calories 281, Fat 13 g, Sat. fat 2 g, Fiber 6 g, Carbs 11 g, Sugars 6 g, Protein 30 g, Sodium 369 mg

Caprese Chicken Hasselback Style

Preparation time: 10 minutes
Cooking time: 30 minutes
Servings: 2

INGREDIENTS:

- ✓ 2 (8 oz. or 226.7g each) skinless chicken breasts, boneless
- ✓ ½ tsp. salt
- ✓ ½ tsp. ground pepper
- ✓ 1 sliced tomato
- ✓ 3 oz. or 85g fresh mozzarella, halved and sliced
- ✓ ¼ c. prepared pesto
- ✓ 8 c. broccoli florets
- ✓ 2 tbsps. olive oil

DIRECTIONS:

1. Set your oven to 375 F/190 C and coat a rimmed baking sheet with cooking spray.
2. Make crosswire cuts at half inches in the chicken breasts. Sprinkle ¼ teaspoons of pepper and salt on them. Fill the cuts with mozzarella slices and tomato alternatively. Brush both the chicken breasts with pesto and put it on the baking sheet.

3. Mix broccoli, oil, salt, and pepper in a bowl. Put this mixture on one side of the baking sheet.
4. Bake till the broccoli is tender, and the chicken is not pink in the center. Cut each of the breasts in half and serve.

NUTRITION: Calories 355 Fat 19 g, Sat. fat 6 g, Fiber 3 g, Carbs 4 g, Sugars 3 g, Protein 38 g, Sodium 634

Grilled Calamari with Lemon Juice

Preparation time: 10 minutes
Cooking time: 15 **minutes**
Servings: 2

INGREDIENTS:

- ¼ c. dried cranberries
- ¼ c. extra virgin olive oil
- ¼ c. olive oil
- ¼ c. sliced almonds
- 1/3 c. fresh lemon juice
- ¾ c. blueberries
- 1 ½ lbs. or 700 g. cleaned calamari tube
- 1 granny smith apple, sliced thinly
- 2 tbsps. apple cider vinegar
- 6 c. fresh spinach
- Grated pepper
- Sea salt

DIRECTIONS:

1. In a medium bowl, mix lemon juice, apple cider vinegar, and extra virgin olive oil to make a sauce. Season with pepper and salt to taste and mix well.

2. Turn on the grill to medium fire and let the grates heat up for 1-2 minutes.
3. In a separate bowl, add in olive oil and the calamari tube. Season calamari generously with pepper and salt.
4. Place calamari onto heated grate and grill for 2-3 minutes each side or until opaque.
5. Meanwhile, combine almonds, cranberries, blueberries, spinach, and the thinly sliced apple in a large salad bowl. Toss to mix.
6. Remove cooked calamari from grill and transfer on a chopping board. Cut into ¼-inch thick rings and throw into the salad bowl.
7. Sprinkle with already prepared sauce. Toss well to coat and serve.

NUTRITION: Calories 567, Fat 24 g, Sat. fat 5 g, Fiber 2 g, Carbs 30.6 g, Sugars 1 g, Protein 54.8 g, Sodium 320 mg

Bacon-Wrapped Chicken

Preparation time: 10 minutes

Cooking time: 50 minutes

Servings: **2**

INGREDIENTS:

- ✓ 4 slices Bacon
- ✓ Salt
- ✓ Pepper
- ✓ 4 oz. or 113 g. Cheddar Cheese, grated
- ✓ 2 Chicken Breasts
- ✓ Paprika to taste
- ✓ 2 tbsps. lemon or orange fresh juice

DIRECTIONS:

1. Heat the oven to 350 F/ 176 C.
2. Place chicken breasts into a medium bowl and season with salt, pepper, paprika, and fresh juice.
3. Replace chicken breasts to a baking pan.
4. Add cheese on top and place bacon slices over chicken breasts.
5. Place the baking pan to the oven for 45 minutes.
6. Take away from the oven your dish and the double-meat meal are ready to be served.

7. Note: If you want to get extra crispy bacon, place your cooked breasts covered with cheese and bacon on a grill or skillet and sauté for 2 minutes on each side.

NUTRITION: Calories 206, Fat 8 g, Sat. fat 3.7 g, Fiber 0 g, Carbs 1.6 g, Sugars 1.6 g, Protein 30 g, Sodium 302 mg

Broccoli Pesto Spaghetti

Preparation time: 10 minutes

Cooking time: 20 minutes

Servings: 2

INGREDIENTS:

- 8 oz. or 226.7g spaghetti
- 1 lb. or 450g broccoli, cut into florets
- 2 tbsps. olive oil
- 4 garlic cloves, chopped
- 4 basil leaves
- 2 tbsps. blanched almonds
- 1 juiced lemon
- Salt and pepper

DIRECTIONS:

1. For the pesto, combine the broccoli, oil, garlic, basil, lemon juice and almonds in a blender and pulse until well mixed and smooth.
2. Set spaghetti in a pot, add salt and pepper. Cook until al dente for about 8 minutes. Drain well.
3. Mix the warm spaghetti with the broccoli pesto and serve.

NUTRITION: Calories 284, Fat 10.2 g, Sat. fat 3 g, Fiber 10 g, Carbs 40.2 g, Sugar 6 g, Protein 10.4 g, Sodium 421 mg

Creamy Chicken Breasts

Preparation time: 10 minutes

Cooking time: 12 minutes

Servings: 4

INGREDIENTS:

- ✓ 4 chicken breasts, skinless and boneless
- ✓ 1 tbsp basil pesto
- ✓ 1 1/2 tbsp cornstarch
- ✓ 1/4 cup roasted red peppers, chopped
- ✓ 1/3 cup heavy cream
- ✓ 1 tsp Italian seasoning
- ✓ 1 tsp garlic, minced
- ✓ 1 cup chicken broth
- ✓ Pepper
- ✓ Salt

DIRECTIONS:

1. Add chicken into the instant pot. Season chicken with Italian seasoning, pepper, and salt. Sprinkle with garlic. Pour broth over chicken. Seal pot with lid and cook on high for 8 minutes.
2. Once done, allow to release pressure naturally for 5 minutes then release remaining using quick

release. Remove lid. Transfer chicken on a plate and clean the instant pot.
3. Set instant pot on sauté mode. Add heavy cream, pesto, cornstarch, and red pepper to the pot and stir well and cook for 3-4 minutes.
4. Return chicken to the pot and coat well with the sauce. Serve and enjoy.

NUTRITION: Calories 341 Fat 15.2 g Carbohydrates 4.4 g Protein 43.8 g

Cheese Garlic Chicken & Potatoes

Preparation time: 10 minutes
Cooking time: 13 minutes
Servings: 4

INGREDIENTS:

- ✓ 2 lb. chicken breasts, skinless, boneless, cut into chunks
- ✓ 1 tbsp olive oil
- ✓ 3/4 cup chicken broth
- ✓ 1 tbsp Italian seasoning
- ✓ 1 tbsp garlic powder
- ✓ 1 tsp garlic, minced
- ✓ 1 1/2 cup parmesan cheese, shredded
- ✓ 1 lb. potatoes, chopped
- ✓ Pepper
- ✓ Salt

DIRECTIONS:

1. Add oil into the inner pot of instant pot and set the pot on sauté mode. Add chicken and cook until browned. Add remaining ingredients except for cheese and stir well.

2. Seal pot with lid and cook on high for 8 minutes. Once done, release pressure using quick release. Remove lid. Top with cheese and cover with lid for 5 minutes or until cheese is melted. Serve and enjoy.

NUTRITION: Calories 674 Fat 29 g Carbohydrates 21.4 g Protein 79.7 g

Easy Chicken Scampi

Preparation time: 10 minutes
Cooking time: 25 minutes
Servings: 4

INGREDIENTS:

- ✓ 3 chicken breasts, skinless, boneless, and sliced
- ✓ 1 tsp garlic, minced
- ✓ 1 tbsp Italian seasoning
- ✓ 2 cups chicken broth
- ✓ 1 bell pepper, sliced
- ✓ 1/2 onion, sliced
- ✓ Pepper, Salt

DIRECTIONS:

1. Add chicken into the instant pot and top with remaining ingredients. Seal pot with lid and cook on high for 25 minutes. Once done, release pressure using quick release. Remove lid.
2. Remove chicken from pot and shred using a fork. Return shredded chicken to the pot and stir well. Serve over cooked whole grain pasta and top with cheese.

NUTRITION: Calories 254 Fat 9.9 g Carbohydrates 4.6 g Protein 34.6 g

Protein Packed Chicken Bean Rice

Preparation time: 10 minutes
Cooking time: 15 minutes
Servings: 6

INGREDIENTS:

- ✓ 1 lb. chicken breasts, skinless, boneless, and cut into chunks
- ✓ 14 oz can cannellini beans, rinsed and drained
- ✓ 4 cups chicken broth
- ✓ 2 cups brown rice
- ✓ 1 tbsp Italian seasoning
- ✓ 1 small onion, chopped
- ✓ 1 tbsp garlic, chopped
- ✓ 1 tbsp olive oil
- ✓ Pepper
- ✓ Salt

DIRECTIONS:

1. Add oil into the inner pot of instant pot and set the pot on sauté mode. Add garlic and onion and sauté for 3 minutes. Add remaining ingredients and stir everything well.

2. Seal pot with a lid and select manual and set timer for 12 minutes. Once done, release pressure using quick release. Remove lid. Stir well and serve.

NUTRITION: Calories 494 Fat 11.3 g Carbohydrates 61.4 g Protein 34.2 g

Pesto Vegetable Chicken

Preparation time: 10 minutes
Cooking time: 25 minutes
Servings: 4

INGREDIENTS:

- ✓ 1 1/2 lb. chicken thighs, skinless, boneless, and cut into pieces
- ✓ 1/2 cup chicken broth
- ✓ 1/4 cup fresh parsley, chopped
- ✓ 2 cups cherry tomatoes, halved
- ✓ 1 cup basil pesto
- ✓ 3/4 lb. asparagus, trimmed and cut in half
- ✓ 2/3 cup sun-dried tomatoes, drained and chopped
- ✓ 2 tbsp olive oil
- ✓ Pepper
- ✓ Salt

DIRECTIONS:

1. Add oil into the inner pot of instant pot and set the pot on sauté mode. Add chicken and sauté for 5 minutes. Add remaining ingredients except for tomatoes and stir well.

2. Seal pot with a lid and select manual and set timer for 15 minutes. Once done, release pressure using quick release. Remove lid.
3. Add tomatoes and stir well. Again, seal the pot and select manual and set timer for 5 minutes. Release pressure using quick release. Remove lid. Stir well and serve.

NUTRITION: Calories 459 Fat 20.5 g Carbohydrates 14.9 g Protein 9.2 g

Greek Chicken Rice

Preparation time: 10 minutes
Cooking time: 14 minutes
Servings: 4

INGREDIENTS:

- 3 chicken breasts, skinless, boneless, and cut into chunks
- 1/4 fresh parsley, chopped
- 1 zucchini, sliced
- 2 bell peppers, chopped
- 1 cup rice, rinsed and drained
- 1 1/2 cup chicken broth
- 1 tbsp oregano
- 3 tbsp fresh lemon juice
- 1 tbsp garlic, minced
- 1 onion, diced
- 2 tbsp olive oil
- Pepper
- Salt

DIRECTIONS:

1. Add oil into the inner pot of instant pot and set the pot on sauté mode. Add onion and chicken and cook for 5 minutes. Add rice, oregano, lemon juice, garlic, broth, pepper, and salt and stir everything well.

2. Seal pot with lid and cook on high for 4 minutes. Once done, release pressure using quick release. Remove lid. Add parsley, zucchini, and bell peppers and stir well.

3. Seal pot again with lid and select manual and set timer for 5 minutes. Release pressure using quick release. Remove lid. Stir well and serve.

NUTRITION: Calories 500 Fat 16.5 g Carbohydrates 48 g Protein 38.7 g

Flavorful Chicken Tacos

Preparation time: 10 minutes
Cooking time: 10 minutes
Servings: 3

INGREDIENTS:

- 2 chicken breasts, skinless and boneless
- 1 tbsp chili powder
- 1/2 tsp ground cumin
- 1/2 tsp garlic powder
- 1/4 tsp onion powder
- 1/2 tsp paprika
- 4 oz can green chilis, diced
- 1/4 cup chicken broth
- 14 oz can tomato, diced
- Pepper
- Salt

DIRECTIONS:

1. Add all ingredients except chicken into the instant pot and stir well. Add chicken and stir. Seal pot with lid and cook on high for 10 minutes.

2. Once done, allow to release pressure naturally for 5 minutes then release remaining using quick release. Remove lid.

3. Remove chicken from pot and shred using a fork. Return shredded chicken to the pot and stir well. Serve and enjoy.

NUTRITION: Calories 237 Fat 8 g Carbohydrates 10.8 g Protein 30.5 g

Quinoa Chicken Bowls

Preparation time: 10 minutes
Cooking time: 6 minutes
Servings: 4

INGREDIENTS:

- ✓ 1 lb. chicken breasts, skinless, boneless, and cut into chunks
- ✓ 14 oz can chickpeas, drained and rinsed
- ✓ 1 cup olives, pitted and sliced
- ✓ 1 cup cherry tomatoes, halved
- ✓ 1 cucumber, sliced
- ✓ 2 tsp Greek seasoning
- ✓ 1 1/2 cups chicken broth
- ✓ 1 cup quinoa, rinsed and drained
- ✓ Pepper
- ✓ Salt

DIRECTIONS:

1. Add broth and quinoa into the instant pot and stir well. Season chicken with Greek seasoning, pepper, and salt and place into the instant pot.

2. Seal pot with lid and cook on high for 6 minutes. Once done, release pressure using quick release. Remove lid. Stir quinoa and chicken mixture well.
3. Add remaining ingredients and stir everything well. Serve immediately and enjoy it.

NUTRITION: Calories 566 Fat 16.4 g Carbohydrates 57.4 g Protein 46.8 g

Quick Chicken with Mushrooms

Preparation time: 10 minutes
Cooking time: 22 minutes
Servings: 6

INGREDIENTS:

- 2 lb. chicken breasts, skinless and boneless
- 1/2 cup heavy cream
- 1/3 cup water
- 3/4 lb. mushrooms, sliced
- 3 tbsp olive oil
- 1 tsp Italian seasoning
- Pepper
- Salt

DIRECTIONS:

1. Add oil into the inner pot of instant pot and set the pot on sauté mode. Season chicken with Italian seasoning, pepper, and salt.
2. Add chicken to the pot and sauté for 5 minutes. Remove chicken from pot and set aside. Add mushrooms and sauté for 5 minutes or until mushrooms are lightly brown.

3. Return chicken to the pot. Add water and stir well. Seal pot with a lid and select manual and set timer for 12 minutes.
4. Once done, release pressure using quick release. Remove lid. Remove chicken from pot and place on a plate.
5. Set pot on sauté mode. Add heavy cream and stir well and cook for 5 minutes. Pour mushroom sauce over chicken and serve.

NUTRITION: Calories 396 Fat 22.3 g Carbohydrates 2.2 g Protein 45.7 g

Herb Garlic Chicken

Preparation time: 10 minutes
Cooking time: 12 minutes
Servings: 8

INGREDIENTS:

- 4 lb. chicken breasts, skinless and boneless
- 1 tbsp garlic powder
- 2 tbsp dried Italian herb mix
- 2 tbsp olive oil
- 1/4 cup chicken stock
- Pepper, Salt

DIRECTIONS:

1. Coat chicken with oil and season with dried herb, garlic powder, pepper, and salt. Place chicken into the instant pot. Pour stock over the chicken. Seal pot with a lid and select manual and set timer for 12 minutes.
2. Once done, allow to release pressure naturally for 5 minutes then release remaining using quick release. Remove lid. Shred chicken using a fork and serve.

NUTRITION: Calories 502 Fat 20.8 g Carbohydrates 7.8 g Protein 66.8 g

The Mediterranean Diet Cookbook: Pork, Beef and Poultry Recipes

Flavorful Mediterranean Chicken

Preparation time: 10 minutes

Cooking time: 20 minutes

Servings: 8

INGREDIENTS:

- ✓ 2 lb. chicken thighs
- ✓ 1/2 cup olives
- ✓ 28 oz can tomato, diced
- ✓ 1 1/2 tsp dried oregano
- ✓ 2 tsp dried parsley
- ✓ 1/2 tsp ground coriander powder
- ✓ 1/4 tsp chili pepper
- ✓ 1 tsp onion powder
- ✓ 1 tsp paprika
- ✓ 2 cups onion, chopped
- ✓ 2 tbsp olive oil
- ✓ Pepper
- ✓ Salt

DIRECTIONS:

1. Add oil into the inner pot of instant pot and set the pot on sauté mode. Add chicken and cook until browned. Transfer chicken on a plate. Add onion and sauté for 5 minutes.
2. Add all spices, tomatoes, and salt and cook for 2-3 minutes. Return chicken to the pot and stir everything well. Seal pot with lid and cook on high for 8 minutes.
3. Once done, release pressure using quick release. Remove lid. Add olives and stir well. Serve and enjoy.

NUTRITION: Calories 292 Fat 13 g Carbohydrates 8.9 g Protein 34.3 g

Artichoke Olive Chicken

Preparation time: 10 minutes
Cooking time: 8 minutes
Servings: 6

INGREDIENTS:

- ✓ 2 1/2 lb. chicken breasts, skinless and boneless
- ✓ 14 oz can artichokes
- ✓ 1/2 cup olives, pitted
- ✓ 3/4 cup prunes
- ✓ 1 tbsp capers
- ✓ 1 1/2 tbsp garlic, chopped
- ✓ 3 tbsp red wine vinegar
- ✓ 2 tsp dried oregano
- ✓ 1/3 cup wine
- ✓ Pepper
- ✓ Salt

DIRECTIONS:

1. Add all ingredients except chicken into the instant pot and stir well. Add chicken and mix well. Seal pot with lid and cook on high for 8 minutes.

2. Once done, allow to release pressure naturally for 10 minutes then release remaining using quick release. Remove lid. Serve and enjoy.

NUTRITION: Calories 472 Fat 15.5 g Carbohydrates 22.7 g Protein 57.6 g

Easy Chicken Piccata

Preparation time: 10 minutes
Cooking time: 41 minutes
Servings: 6

INGREDIENTS:

- ✓ 8 chicken thighs, bone-in, and skin-on
- ✓ 2 tbsp fresh parsley, chopped
- ✓ 1 tbsp olive oil
- ✓ 3 tbsp capers
- ✓ 2 tbsp fresh lemon juice
- ✓ 1/2 cup chicken broth
- ✓ 1/4 cup dry white wine
- ✓ 1 tbsp garlic, minced

DIRECTIONS:

1. Add oil into the inner pot of instant pot and set the pot on sauté mode. Add garlic and sauté for 1 minute. Add wine and cook for 5 minutes or until wine reduced by half.
2. Add lemon juice and broth and stir well. Add chicken and seal pot with the lid and select manual and set a timer for 30 minutes.

3. Once done, release pressure using quick release. Remove lid. Remove chicken from pot and place on a baking tray. Broil chicken for 5 minutes. Add capers and stir well. Garnish with parsley and serve.

NUTRITION: Calories 406 Fat 17 g Carbohydrates 1.2 g Protein 57 g

Garlic Thyme Chicken Drumsticks

Preparation time: 10 minutes
Cooking time: 18 minutes
Servings: 4

INGREDIENTS:

- 8 chicken drumsticks, skin-on
- 2 tbsp balsamic vinegar
- 2/3 cup can tomato, diced
- 6 garlic cloves
- 1 tsp lemon zest, grated
- 1 tsp dried thyme
- 1/4 tsp red pepper flakes
- 1 1/2 onions, cut into wedges
- 1 tbsp olive oil
- Pepper
- Salt

DIRECTIONS:

1. Add oil into the inner pot of instant pot and set the pot on sauté mode. Add onion and 1/2 tsp salt and sauté for 2-3 minutes.

2. Add chicken, garlic, lemon zest, red pepper flakes, and thyme and mix well. Add vinegar and tomatoes and stir well.
3. Seal pot with lid and cook on high for 15 minutes. Once done, release pressure using quick release. Remove lid. Stir well and serve.

NUTRITION: Calories 220 Fat 8.9 g Carbohydrates 7.8 g Protein 26.4 g

Tender Chicken & Mushrooms

Preparation time: 10 minutes

Cooking time: 21 minutes

Servings: 6

INGREDIENTS:

- ✓ 1 lb. chicken breasts, skinless, boneless, & cut into 1-inch pieces
- ✓ 1/4 cup olives, sliced
- ✓ 2 oz feta cheese, crumbled
- ✓ 1/4 cup sherry
- ✓ 1 cup chicken broth
- ✓ 1 tsp Italian seasoning
- ✓ 12 oz mushrooms, sliced
- ✓ 2 celery stalks, diced
- ✓ 1 tsp garlic, minced
- ✓ 1/2 cup onion, chopped
- ✓ 2 tbsp olive oil
- ✓ Pepper
- ✓ Salt

DIRECTIONS:

1. Add oil into the inner pot of instant pot and set the pot on sauté mode. Add mushrooms, celery, garlic, and onion and sauté for 5-7 minutes.
2. Add chicken, Italian seasoning, pepper, and salt and stir well and cook for 4 minutes. Add sherry and broth and stir well. Seal pot with lid and cook on high for 10 minutes.
3. Once done, allow to release pressure naturally for 10 minutes then release remaining using quick release. Remove lid. Add olives and feta cheese and stir well. Serve and enjoy.

NUTRITION: Calories 244 Fat 13.5 g Carbohydrates 4.1 g Protein 26 g

Delicious Chicken Casserole

Preparation time: 10 minutes
Cooking time: 20 minutes
Servings: 4

INGREDIENTS:

- ✓ 1 lb. chicken breasts, skinless, boneless, & cubed
- ✓ 2 tsp paprika
- ✓ 3 tbsp tomato paste
- ✓ 1 cup chicken stock
- ✓ 4 tomatoes, chopped
- ✓ 1 small eggplant, chopped
- ✓ 1 tbsp Italian seasoning
- ✓ 2 bell pepper, sliced
- ✓ 1 onion, sliced
- ✓ 1 tbsp garlic, minced
- ✓ 1 tbsp olive oil
- ✓ Pepper
- ✓ Salt

DIRECTIONS:

1. Add oil into the inner pot of instant pot and set the pot on sauté mode. Season chicken with pepper

and salt and add into the instant pot. Cook chicken until lightly golden brown.
2. Remove chicken from pot and place on a plate. Add garlic and onion and sauté until onion is softened about 3-5 minutes.
3. Return chicken to the pot. Pour remaining ingredients over chicken and stir well. Seal pot with lid and cook on high for 10 minutes.
4. Once done, release pressure using quick release. Remove lid. Stir well and serve.

NUTRITION: Calories 356 Fat 13.9 g Carbohydrates 22.7 g Protein 36.9 g

Moroccan Chicken

Preparation time: 10 minutes
Cooking time: 25 minutes
Servings: 6

INGREDIENTS:

- 2 lb. chicken breasts, cut into chunks
- 1/2 tsp cinnamon
- 1 tsp turmeric
- 1/2 tsp ginger
- 1 tsp cumin
- 2 tbsp Dijon mustard
- 1 tbsp molasses
- 1 tbsp honey
- 2 tbsp tomato paste
- 5 garlic cloves, chopped
- 2 onions, cut into quarters
- 2 green bell peppers, cut into strips
- 2 red bell peppers, cut into strips
- 2 cups olives, pitted
- 1 lemon, peeled and sliced
- 2 tbsp olive oil

- ✓ Pepper
- ✓ Salt

DIRECTIONS:

1. Add oil into the inner pot of instant pot and set the pot on sauté mode. Add chicken and sauté for 5 minutes. Add remaining ingredients and stir everything well.
2. Seal pot with a lid and select manual and set timer for 20 minutes. Once done, release pressure using quick release. Remove lid. Stir well and serve.

NUTRITION: Calories 446 Fat 21.2 g Carbohydrates 18.5 g Protein 45.8 g

Flavorful Cafe Rio Chicken

Preparation time: 10 minutes

Cooking time: 12 minutes

Servings: 6

INGREDIENTS:

- ✓ 2 lb. chicken breasts, skinless and boneless
- ✓ 1/2 cup chicken stock
- ✓ 2 1/2 tbsp ranch seasoning
- ✓ 1/2 tbsp ground cumin
- ✓ 1/2 tbsp chili powder
- ✓ 1/2 tbsp garlic, minced
- ✓ 2/3 cup Italian dressing
- ✓ Pepper
- ✓ Salt

DIRECTIONS:

1. Add chicken into the instant pot. Mix together remaining ingredients and pour over chicken. Seal pot with a lid and select manual and set timer for 12 minutes.
2. Once done, allow to release pressure naturally for 10 minutes then release remaining using quick

release. Remove lid. Shred the chicken using a fork and serve.

NUTRITION: Calories 382 Fat 18.9 g Carbohydrates 3.6 g Protein 44.1 g

Zesty Veggie Chicken

Preparation time: 10 minutes
Cooking time: 5 minutes
Servings: 4

INGREDIENTS:

- ✓ 1 lb. chicken tender, skinless, boneless and cut into chunks
- ✓ 10 oz of frozen vegetables
- ✓ 1/3 cup zesty Italian dressing
- ✓ 1/2 tsp Italian seasoning
- ✓ 1 cup fried onions
- ✓ 2/3 cup rice
- ✓ 1 cup chicken broth
- ✓ Pepper
- ✓ Salt

DIRECTIONS:

1. Add all ingredients except vegetables into the instant pot. Meanwhile, cook frozen vegetables in microwave according to packet instructions.
2. Seal pot with lid and cook on high for 5 minutes. Once done, allow to release pressure naturally for

10 minutes then release remaining using quick release. Remove lid.
3. Add cooked vegetables and stir well. Serve and enjoy.

NUTRITION: Calories 482 Fat 15.9 g Carbohydrates 40.5 g Protein 38.3 g

Lightning Source UK Ltd.
Milton Keynes UK
UKHW021836220621
385995UK00002B/223